MUSCLEMAG
INTERNATIONAL

THE
BOTTOM
LINE

YOUR FASTEST WAY TO A SEXY BUTT

BY ROBERT KENNEDY & DWAYNE HINES II

Copyright © 2000 By Robert Kennedy

All rights reserved including the right to reproduce
this book or portions thereof in any form whatsoever.

Published by MuscleMag International
5775 McLaughlin Road
Mississauga, ON
L5R 3P7

Designed by Jackie Kydyk
Edited by Matt Lamperd

Canadian Cataloguing in Publication Data

Kennedy, Robert, 1938-
   The bottom line:your fastest way to a sexy butt

ISBN 1-55210-022-7

   1. Exercise for women. 2.Buttocks. I.Hines,
Dwayne, 1961- II.Title.

GV508.K45 2000   646.7'5   C00-901321-0

Distributed in Canada by
CANBOOK Distribution Services
1220 Nicholson Road
Newmarket, ON
L3Y 7V1
800-399-6858

Distributed in the States by
BookWorld Services
1933 Whitfield Park Loop
Sarasota, FL 34243

Printed in Canada

Table of Contents

INTRODUCTION

What concerns you the most about your appearance? Your hair? Your lips? Nose? For a lot of women, the top area of concern is actually the bottom area – the buns and the hips. When it comes down to top priority, the appearance of the buns takes precedence over everything else. And with good reason. Your buttocks and hips define your appearance from the back, as well as from the front.

Your hips and buns can greatly enhance or detract from your overall appearance – depending upon the condition they are in. This area of the physique is a body appearance "multiplier." The muscle groups involved add a positive emphasis to your body if they are trimmed and toned, or decrease your appearance if they are either too flabby or too flat.

Too Flabby or Too Flat?

When it comes to problems with their posteriors, most women automatically think of the "too much" problem – too much size and too much muscle softness (the skin should be soft, but not the muscle, which should be firm). Buns that are too big, or loose and flabby, are a major appearance problem. But there is another problem that some women struggle with that can be just as frustrating – buns and hips that are too flat and tiny. Yes, the buns and hips can be too small in the aesthetic sense. Those who have large hips and buttocks may wish they had this type of problem, but why exchange one problem for another?

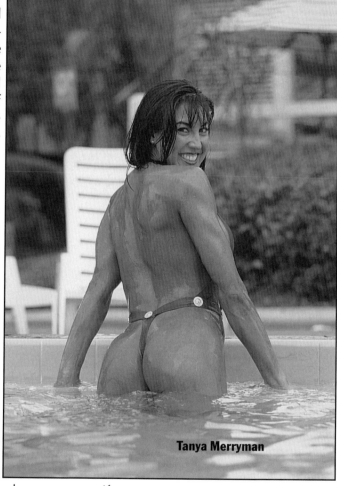

Tanya Merryman

Fortunately, each of these problems can be overcome, if you know what to do for them. *The Bottom Line* addresses these problems and more in the upcoming pages. You can shape beautiful glutes and have trimmer hips. This book will show you how.

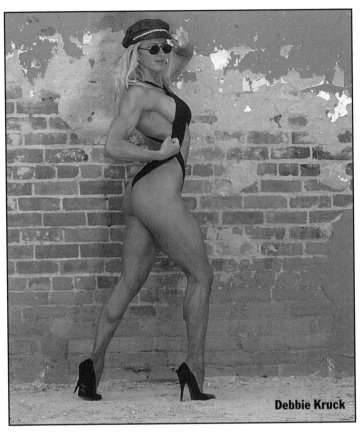

Debbie Kruck

Several Essential Factors

When it comes to shaping a pair of beautiful buns and trim hips, there is no one magic trick that will instantly transform your posterior overnight. Although there are many fad gadgets on the market for supposedly shaping the hips and buttocks instantly, the truth is, no changes to the body are instantaneous. The body takes time to be re-shaped. And it takes a lot of effort. Yes, significant changes are possible, but they are not possible in two weeks. You cannot completely "transform your buns in 14 days." If you accept this fact, it will help you avoid the expectation trap. Many people fall prey to this advertising scheme – where the media promises instantaneous changes if you just buy this product or that service.

There are several factors that need to be employed to successfully shape the hips and buns, and time needs to be allowed to accomplish this task. Using all of the major factors together will help you achieve the shape that you want much more readily than if you use only one element.

Your Fastest Way To A Sexy Butt

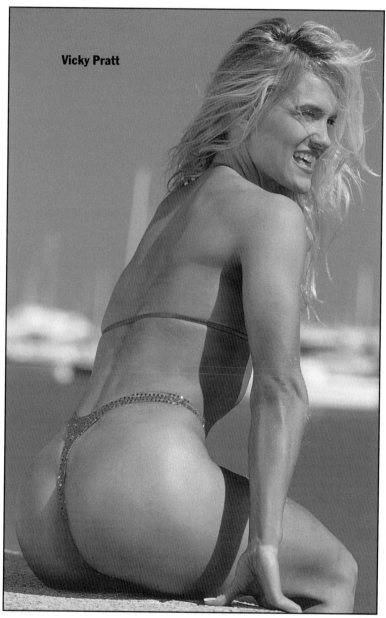

Vicky Pratt

Allow Yourself Time to Change

By realizing that it is not possible to re-shape your body shape in a couple of weeks, you take the pressure off of yourself to make things happen "today". This is the best way to work with the body in changing its shape. Instead of fighting any type of instant change – it likes the status quo. In order to make some necessary changes happen smoothly, use a gradual approach. A gradual approach takes a little

Your Fastest Way To A Sexy Butt

longer but the results are long-lasting. And that is what you want. What good is looking great for only a few days? Real change takes more time but endures. This applies to your physique and in turn to your hips and buns.

Shape

What is meant by the terminology of "shaping" your body is actually "reshaping" your body. Your body already has shape – and that shape is good or bad. This condition of this shape is of course subjective – but most people have a good idea of what looks hot in the area of the hips and buns. And the "good shape" consists of a trim (but not too tiny) area with good firm muscle tone. However, knowing what good posterior shape is and achieving it are two different things. And most women want to change – to "upgrade" – the shape of their hips and buns.

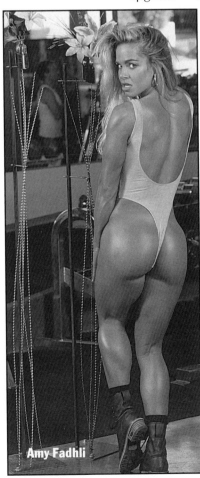

Amy Fadhli

The shape of your body changes a little bit every few weeks and only three possibilities exist – you are either getting better, holding even, or getting worse. For the vast majority of people (who generally are mostly sedentary), the shape of their body takes a gradual decline over the years. Each year their muscle tone loses a little bit of ground, and fat gains ground. This does not have to occur! Research has indicated that people in their seventies who work out are as strong or stronger than people in their twenties who don't exercise. Working out, along with the supporting elements of diet and a healthy lifestyle, provides the supreme manner in which to fight the loss of muscle tone and shape in your body. By using specific factors (working out, diet, stretching etc.), the shape of the human physique can be altered in a positive way. *The Bottom Line* will provide you with the direction on what to do and how to do it – all you have to do is apply the tips and techniques to your own body. The shape of the human body will yield to your commands if you are consistent in using the right techniques to change it. What are they? Read on to find out!

Your Fastest Way To A Sexy Butt

Chapter One

SUPER SPECIFIC SHAPE EXERCISES

Exercise works best when it is used in a specific manner. For instance, cardiovascular/respiratory or aerobic exercise is primarily intended to increase the health of the body – particularly the heart and lungs. Aerobic exercise is also a great way to burn off body fat. Strength/shape exercise is primarily intended to increase the muscle tone, strength and shape of your body. Each of these exercises provide other secondary benefits, but each has its specific primary benefit. The first step in body shaping success is finding the right tool to use. For shaping the buns and hips, there are a variety of tools but none is as important as specific shape exercise. Other exercise tools such as aerobics and nutrition are part of the bun/hip shaping program and will be discussed in upcoming chapters. If you want to positively change the shape of your posterior it is crucial that you use the best tool – specific shape exercises.

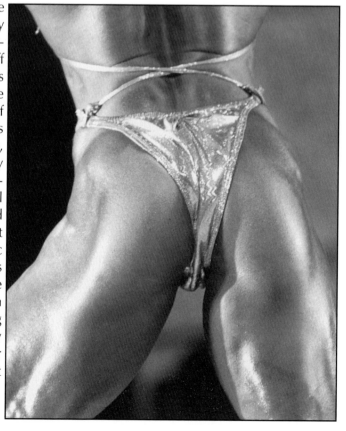

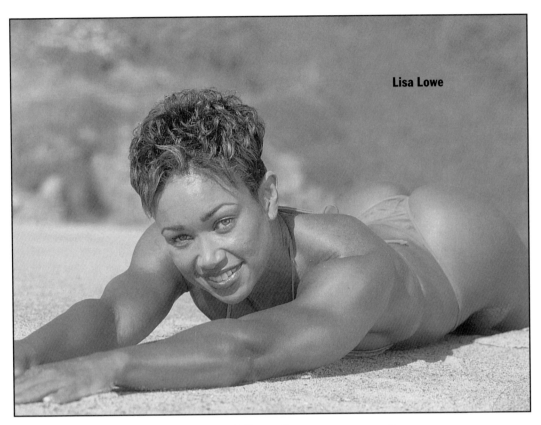

Lisa Lowe

Specific Shape Exercises

Specific shape exercises allow you to target the precise area that you want to work on. Instead of messing around with largely unproductive general exercises you can get right to the point of the matter – your posterior. And specific shape exercises produce significant results if they are used consistently. Specific shape exercises are used to hit the hips and buns hard, making this area respond with more muscle tone and overall tightness.

Shape Exercises & Muscle Tone

The exercises that work on the hip/bun area do so by increasing the muscle tone of the hips and buns. Muscles by their very nature are firm. The body is made in such a manner that muscles are firm; fat is loose.

As mentioned earlier, another equally important factor is shape. The more you tone your muscles, the more you positively alter the shape of your physique. Shape is also a consideration for those who have buns and hips that

Your Fastest Way To A Sexy Butt

are too thin. When muscle tone is added to skinny hips and flat buns, they gain a much better shape, having nice curves instead of just straight lines.

The key to overcome both flabby buns and flat buns is to build up the muscle tone of the body, particularly in this area of the hips and buns. Specific shaping exercises enable you to do exactly that. In addition to the number one goal of building up muscle tone, specific shaping exercises also have a fantastic secondary benefit – they burn off bodyfat. It is the combination of increasing the muscle tone and burning off bodyfat that really makes the hips and buns significantly change in a positive manner. The manner in which specific shaping exercise burns off more of your body fat is primarily through a metabolic boost.

Bun Shaping & the Metabolic Boost

Your metabolism is the number one fat-burning factor for the physique. Your body's basal metabolic rate is responsible for as many as 75 percent of the calories used by the body on a daily basis. Burning off calories is how you burn off bodyfat. And since fat is half the problem of the hips and buns (the other half is lack of muscle tone and well-contoured shape) then it is a good idea to take advantage of this high-powered fat burning tool. Shape/strength exercises present a unique way to obtain dual fat burning results from the metabolism.

When you perform shaping/strength exercises you significantly elevate your metabolism. If you perform the shaping exercises intensely, your metabolism stays elevated long after the exercise is over. Some studies show that the metabolism stays elevated as long as a full day after intense exercise. Shape/strength exercise boosts your metabolism

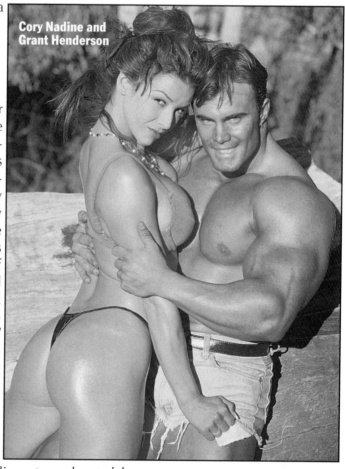

Cory Nadine and Grant Henderson

Your Fastest Way To A Sexy Butt

much more than other forms of exercise like cardio/aerobic or stretching exercise due to the "post-workout burn". The post-workout burn for aerobic training lasts only a very short time after you complete your workout. When you perform aerobic exercise your body primarily burns fat during the exercise and for a few minutes after the exercise. On the other hand, when you perform shape/strength exercise, your body primarily burns carbohydrates during the exercise and fat after the exercise is over. But this fat burning does not stop after a few minutes as it does with aerobic training. Instead, the body continues to burn up fat at a faster pace for hours after the exercise. For this reason shape/strength exercise is fantastic for getting rid of fat. Consider the athletes who perform a lot of shape/strength exercise – the body-builders. These people have super low body fat levels (single digit) and the frequent shape/strength training they do is a major factor in this outcome. You can enjoy similar fat-burning results if you incorporate frequent shape/strength training sessions into your workout program.

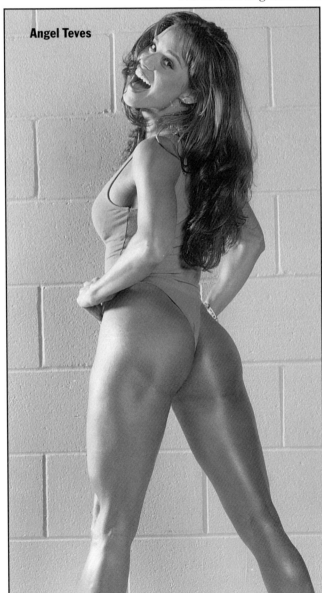

Angel Teves

The "post-workout burn" is not the only fat-burning result that shape/strength exercise produces. The second fat-burning result of shape/strength training is the raised level of metabolic activity even when you are resting. This is the "sedentary burn". The sedentary burn comes about because muscle tissue is more active than fat tissue – even when you are resting. You will burn 30 to 50 more calories every day for each extra pound of muscle you put on because lean body mass takes more energy to sustain than does fat. So if you add five pounds of

Your Fastest Way To A Sexy Butt

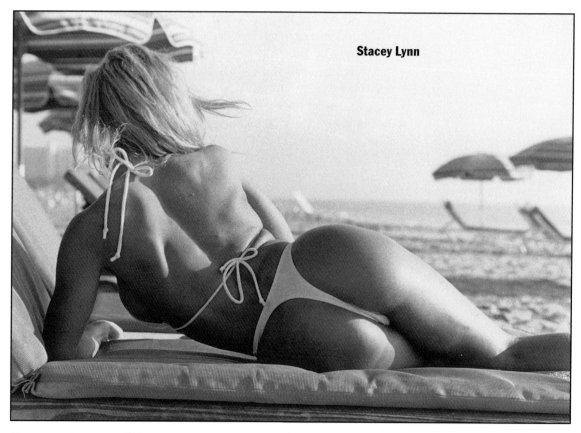

Stacey Lynn

firm muscle, you will burn 150 to 250 more calories every day than you had previously been burning off. The increase in muscle tone really helps you achieve the decrease in bodyfat that you want. That is why adding some muscle tone to your body is such a great way to really re-shape your physique.

Both of the fat-burning results of shape/strength training benefit the shape of your buns and hips because the less fat this area has (up to a point) the better it looks. A lean posterior looks great – provided it has some muscle tone to give it nice, controlled curves.

Controlled Curves

One of the crucial goals to aim at in re-shaping the hips and buns is to create curves – controlled curves. Many women have curves in this region but they are not necessarily controlled curves! Uncontrolled curves in the posterior area are the lament of many people. Buns that are not under control are often "droopy" (too soft in the sense

Your Fastest Way To A Sexy Butt

of muscle tone, not skin quality). The way to bring about contour control for the hips and buns comes through specific shape/strength training. Control means having the curves and shape that you want to have in your hips and buns.

Burning fat off your behind is a secondary result of shape/strength training. The primary result is the control and enhancement of the muscle tone.

There are a variety of excellent exercises you can do to increase the muscle tone in your tail-side. The first exercise is a combination exercise – it works both the hips and buns.

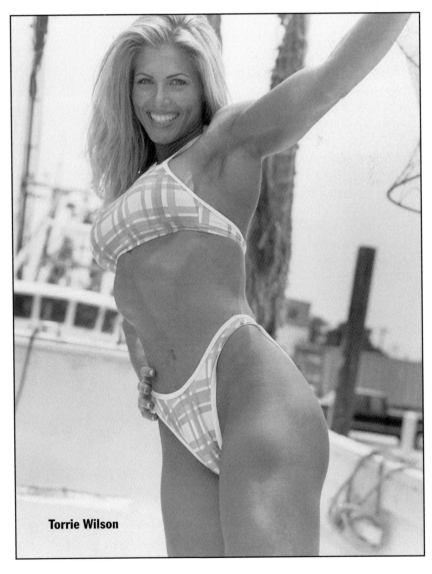

Torrie Wilson

Your Fastest Way To A Sexy Butt

The Hot Hyperextension

This exercise is fantastic because it places the workout spotlight right on your buns and hips (and it also works the small of your lower back to boot). The hyperextension can be performed with your body weight only, which allows you to build muscle tone and not mass. Your body will supply sufficient resistance, and you can increase the repetition range as far as you want to.

Many gyms and health clubs have this excellent piece of equipment as it is a fitness favorite. If you want your own you can obtain one through a sporting goods store or fitness equipment company. It can also be ordered via fitness catalog companies.

The way to perform the hyperextension movement is by taking a prone (and elevated) position on the hyperextension machine. This will put your legs in a braced position just below the calf, and at the thighs. From the elevated prone position you are in (your upper torso appears to be floating in the air) you place your hands behind your head and lower your upper body downward slowly. At the bottom of the movement your head will be just above the floor. From

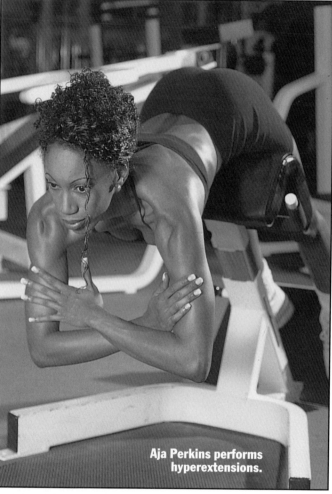

Aja Perkins performs hyperextensions.

this position (45 degree downward) you raise your upper body (the lower body remains braced and motionless) back up to a position where your entire body is parallel with the floor. Your buns, hips, and lower back do the brunt of the work in elevating your upper body back up to a prone position. You can increase the involvement of your buns and hips by specifically contracting and flexing them hard at the top of the movement for a couple of seconds. As your strength increases in this hip/bun movement over the period of several weeks you can add more repetitions.

Your Fastest Way To A Sexy Butt

Squats

The squat is a controversial exercise. Many people avoid it because it can build the buns up too much. Others think it is great. The bottom line is that squatting with heavy weights will add size to your hips and buns. On the other hand, squatting is very good for improving the muscle tone of not only the legs but also the hips and buns – if you use light weights. When it comes to working on the hips and buns, the rule of thumb is that light squatting is good; heavy squatting is not. Avoid heavy squats and concentrate on lighter squatting movements with higher repetitions. There is one exception which will be addressed in the next chapter – people with flat buns and/or thin hips. Heavier squatting is good if you have this condition. One key in making the movement more effective is to make certain that your back is as straight as possible as you squat. The more you bend forward the more emphasis you put on your buns, so keep your back straight. This

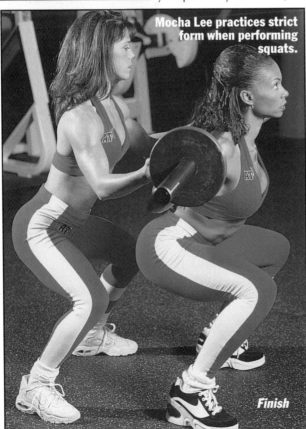

Start

Mocha Lee practices strict form when performing squats.

Finish

will give the buttocks only a minimal role in the movement – which is exactly what you want. Another trick to minimize the overload of the buns in the squat is to take a narrow stance and to place your heels on a raised surface. Don't squat flat-footed; it puts too much emphasis on the buns alone. And don't squat with a wide stance – it also places too much of a load on the buns. The best way to tighten the buns with the squat is to let them take a secondary role instead of a primary role in moving the weight. If you do choose to use the squat, go light, keep your back straight, your stance narrow, and elevate your heels (a couple of inches will do fine).

Your Fastest Way To A Sexy Butt

An excellent squat variation that is favorable for tight buns and hips is the single-leg non-weight squat. This fantastic exercise is performed by squatting down on one leg (balance your body with a hand against the nearest wall) to a point where your thigh is parallel with the floor, and then to come slowly back up. This leg/hip/buns movement will tighten your hips and buns without building them up too much. It is one of the best squatting movements and can be done anywhere without equipment.

Light Stiff-leg Deadlifts

Stiff-leg deadlifts are well known for shaping the hamstrings. They also have a strong secondary effect on the gluteal muscles. You can use them to help you tone up your hips and buns. Grasp a barbell and bend forward, keeping your legs straight except for a little bend in your knees and your back straight. Bend down until the barbell is at the level of your shins, then come back up. Come all the way up (standing straight up), tighten your buns, and repeat. Use a light barbell for this exercise.

Standing Leg Lifts & Back Leg Raises

Now let's take a look at a pair of fantastic specific shaping exercises for the buns and hips – the back leg raise and the standing leg lift. The back leg raise is performed from the prone push-up position. From here one leg is slowly raised four to six inches while the rest of your body is held still. Hold this position and tighten your buns. Repeat with the other side. Perform 10 to 15 repetitions for each buttock. This exercise is great for putting emphasis right on your buttocks – you can really feel them work! And your hips also get involved in the movement.

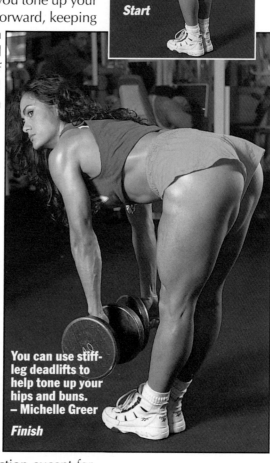

Start

You can use stiff-leg deadlifts to help tone up your hips and buns.
– Michelle Greer

Finish

The standing leg lift is similar in action except for the factor that you are standing instead of laying down. From the standing position bend your upper body forward and brace it on a table ledge or chair. Raise one leg

Your Fastest Way To A Sexy Butt

rearward as high as possible and hold for a second or two at the top of the movement while tightening your buttocks. Repeat with the other side. Both buns and hips are the focus of the work in this movement with the buns getting the primary work load and the hips getting the secondary action.

Floor Raises

A very simple but effective bun/hip exercise are floor raises. Lie face down on the floor and place your hands behind your head (using the torso as support for your body). Raise both your head area and your feet back and up at the same time. Hold this position and squeeze your butt muscles. Lower, and repeat. If you get it right, your body will move from a flat line to a slight arching U-shape, with your torso on the ground and your head and feet arching towards each other.

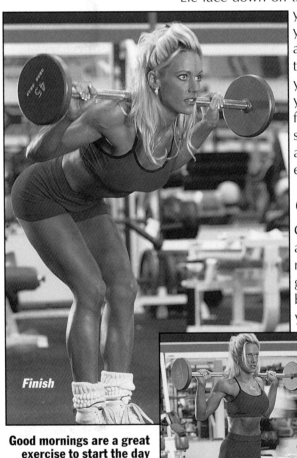

Finish

Good mornings are a great exercise to start the day off with – hence the name. – Brandy Maddron

Start

Good Morning Exercise

Good mornings work your lower back and posterior region. Initially use this movement without weights, then progress onward by placing a very light barbell across your shoulders behind your neck. Do good mornings simply by bending forward at the waist, keeping the legs and back straight. Go down until your back is almost parallel with the floor, then come up slowly. This is a great exercise to start the day off with – hence the name. It also gives your hips and buns a good start.

Hip/Leg Raises

The hip/leg raise is performed from a standing position. Slowly raise one of your legs out to the side of your body as high as possible. Hold for a second, then slowly lower it

Your Fastest Way To A Sexy Butt

down. Repeat on both sides for multiple repetitions. This exercise works your hips well.

Bun Machine

There is a piece of equipment that is made specifically for hitting the buns. This "bun machine" (it goes by a variety of names) can work well for you if you use it right. And the right way to use it is with lighter weights and higher repetitions. Use this machine with the same approach that you use for the squat – don't lift the heavier weights.

Secondary Hip/Bun Support

There are a variety of exercises that work the hips and buns in a secondary manner. That is, their main function is to work another muscle group but in doing so they also involve the tush. A couple of these exercises include the "lunge" and the leg curl. If you are not performing either of these movements in your regular training you might want to consider adding one or both or rotating them in with your other hip/bun exercises to give your fanny an additional boost.

Hip & Bun Exercise

Direct hip and bun exercise is fantastic for effectively tightening your hips and buns. This type of specific shaping exercise will significantly build up your muscle tone and strength in both these areas. When you combine this new muscle tone with a loss of bodyfat in this region (due to the increase in your metabolic rate and decrease of bodyfat from

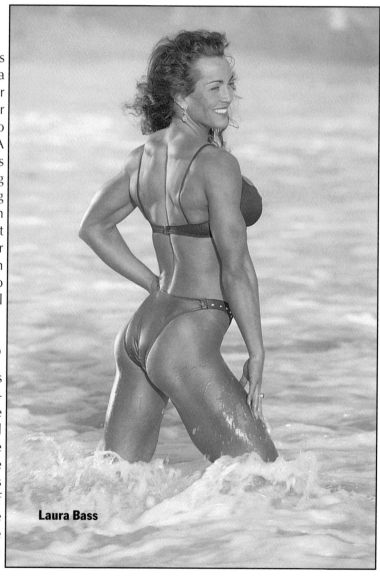

Laura Bass

Your Fastest Way To A Sexy Butt

consistent cardio/aerobic exercise, better diet, increased activity, etc.) your hips and buns will really start to look noticeably more shapely in a positive manner.

Try between one and four sets of the specific shaping exercises for your lower region. Choose at least two exercises from among those listed and get in a good workout. Do each set for as many repetitions as you can. Generally, the higher the repetition count the better. Make sure to do your direct hip/buns training one to three times a week. You do not have to perform all of the exercises listed each time you work out – simply choose a few and do a few sets of each. Don't use the same exercises all of the time – alternate and use a different type once every few workouts. A few possible combinations include:

Light squats
Hyperextensions
Hip/Leg raises
Floor raises

or

Good Mornings
Non-weight one-leg squats
Light stiff-leg deadlifts
Standing leg lifts

If you are short on time you might want to use a modified hip/bun training version:

Hyperextensions
Back leg raises

Remember, some training is always better than no training and a modified hip/bun workout gives you some stimulation for your posterior.

If you train at home and have only minimal equipment a good routine would be:

Non-weight one-leg squats
Standing leg lifts
Back leg raises

These exercises can all be performed without equipment and allow you to get in a good home training workout.

These workout combinations are only sugges- tions and provided as general guidelines – you can make up your own creative hip/bun training schedule. The key point is to get in a few specific hip/bun shaping exercises a week.

Don't perform your training on back-to-back days. Your body needs a certain amount of rest and recuperation – particularly when it comes to building up muscle tone. Take a day or two off between workout sessions. However, don't take too much time off.

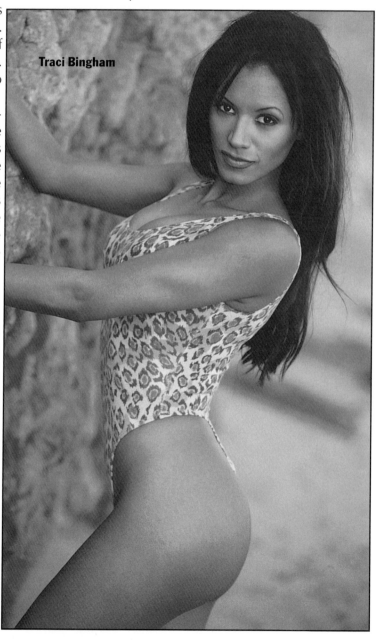

Traci Bingham

Specific shape exercise is important for the hip/bun area because it helps form and shape the muscle tone as it develops. Shape training not only promotes muscle tone; it helps the muscle tone appear in the areas that you want it to – the hips and buns.

Tighten Up!

In addition to the specific shaping exercises, you can make further progress by utilizing direct bun and hip tightening techniques. You can perform this type of hip/bun tightening on a more frequent basis (more frequent than the one to three specific shaping workouts per week). Direct bun/hip tightening is quite simple – you tighten your buns and hips for several repetitions at several times during the day. This involves strongly contracting the muscles in this region for a few seconds, then relaxing

Your Fastest Way To A Sexy Butt

them. This is a very basic way to work this region but many people overlook it. It is easy to do functionally but it really is challenging to the muscles in the hips and buns and they respond by becoming tighter. The key is to get into the habit of taking a couple of seconds to "tighten up" when you get the opportunity during the day. You can do this most anywhere. Just tighten up by clenching your hip and bun muscles as tightly as you can for a couple of seconds, then relax them. Repeat for a few repetitions on several occasions during the day. This direct tightening is easy to perform and yields good results. There are a couple of ways you can enhance this direct tightening. By putting your heel solidly against the floor (this works best where there is carpet) you can get a stronger contraction. And by moving one leg slightly to the rear and side, you can get an even better contraction of the hip/bun area.

Direct tightening can speed up the process of making your hips and buns tighter and muscle toned. Take advantage of this technique for quicker shape results.

Specific shape exercise, along with direct tightening exercise, will work together to help you make significant strides forward in building a nice, shapely tail section. When it comes to shaping the hips and buns, specific shaping exercise is the primary element.

Summary

- Perform specific shaping exercises for the hip and buns 1 to 3 times a week.
- Use higher repetitions (10+) for these muscle groups.
- Perform direct tightening exercise on a consistent daily basis in addition to the specific shaping exercises.

Your Fastest Way To A Sexy Butt

Chapter Two

FILLING OUT FLAT BUNS AND HIPS

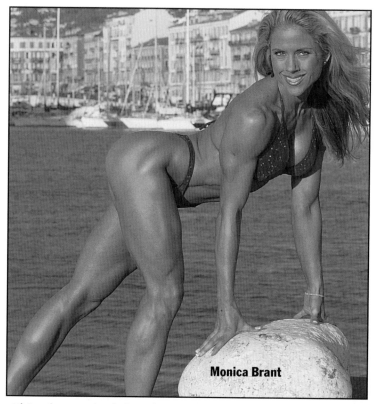

Monica Brant

This chapter is definitely not for everyone. Most people struggle with buns and hips that are more than "filled out". However, there are some people who do have the dilemma of flat buns and skinny hips. Their posterior problem is that they have no real contours in this region and some contours here make the hips and buns look much better. Adding a little size to the buns and hips also makes the rest of your midsection look smaller. Overcoming the "flat bun" problem will help balance the appearance of your middle.

Muscle Contours

When aiming at filling out flat buns and hips, the goal is not just to add size. Extra size may come in the form of fat, and that is not going to look attractive. Instead, the focus needs to be placed on adding size that is based on muscle. Muscle contours really can make your rear view look much better, giving it a sensuous curved appearance. Increasing muscle tone ensures that the contours you add are firm. And as in the previous chapter, it is specific exercise that controls the formation of these curves. Certain specific exercises will bring about definite results. But since the aim of filling out the buns is different than merely increasing the muscle tone (which was the primary goal of the past chapter) the employment of specific bun and hip exercises will be different.

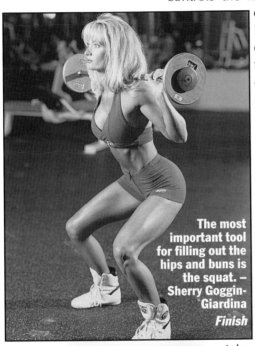

The most important tool for filling out the hips and buns is the squat. –
Sherry Goggin-Giardina

Finish

Super Squat Emphasis

The most important tool for filling out the hips and buns is the squat – particularly when used with heavier weights. Heavier squatting will make the hips and buns start to grow bigger. Many people have experienced significant size increase in the glutes when using heavy squatting on a consistent basis. As you use heavier weight, the hips and buns take over a larger percentage of the workload. With lighter squats, the legs do most of the work. When you go to heavier weights, the gluteals become much more involved, assisting the legs in moving the heavier weight.

Start off your squatting approach with lighter weights, and gradually increase the amount of weight. Don't immediately dive into the deep end of heavy iron use. Slowly build your buns, hips, and legs up to a point where they can handle the heavier challenge. And your body will begin to respond – most likely in a significant manner if you give it some time.

Heavy squatting has another benefit – it really gives the metabolism a strong boost. This means that it will be easier for you to burn off bodyfat, and that insures that the size you add is fat-free.

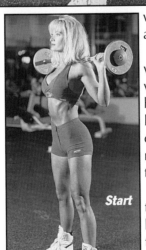

Start

Leg Presses

Leg presses provide benefits that are somewhat similar to the squat. Although not quite as stimulating as squats for the overall lower area, it is a good alternative exercise and can be used for building up your buns if you have access to one.

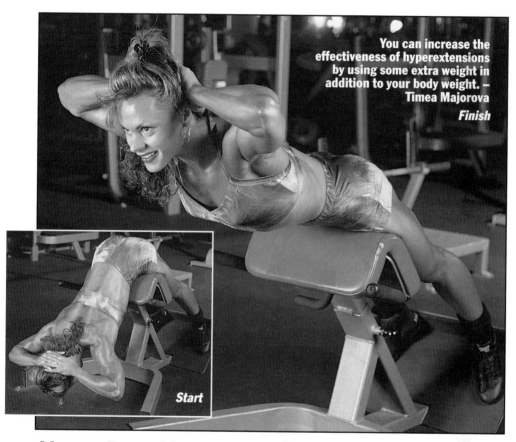

You can increase the effectiveness of hyperextensions by using some extra weight in addition to your body weight. — Timea Majorova

Finish

Start

Heavy Duty Hyperextensions

Hyperextension movements are great for targeting the hips and buns. And you can increase their effectiveness for adding a little size by using some extra weight in addition to your body weight. First get used to the movement by performing it without weight. Then move up to the next level by holding a five pound weight plate behind your head or in front of your chest as you perform the hyperextension movement. Gradually increase the amount of weight that you use and you will gradually stimulate your hips and buns to fill out with contours of muscle.

Your Fastest Way To A Sexy Butt

The Bun Machine

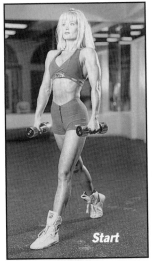

Start

As mentioned in the preceding chapter, the bun machine is a good way to enhance your curves. The caution of the last chapter to use only light weight does not apply if you are trying to fill out your buns and add some size to your hips. Instead of going light, gradually increase the weight stack. Don't be afraid to use quite a bit of weight for this exercise. And once you can handle the weight, keep increasing the repetitions. However, gradually increase both the additional weight and the repetition range to allow your body to adjust to the challenge.

Weighted Mule Kick Backs

Weighted mule kick backs provide yet another exercise tool for overcoming the flat bun/skinny hip syndrome. The regular kick back move is done from a kneeling position with hands and knees on the floor. One leg is lifted up and backwards in a motion similar to a mule kicking (except this is performed with one leg instead of two). To achieve a better effect in promoting new muscle size, put a weighted strap around you ankle. Perform this movement for both sides of your posterior. Start with a very light weight, and gradually work up to a heavier ankle weight. For an even more intense workout, hold your leg in the up position for a few seconds.

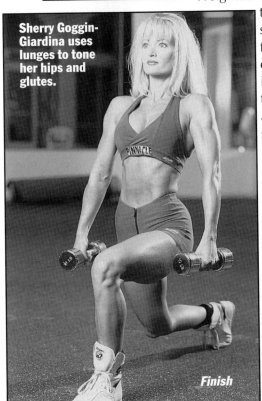

Sherry Goggin-Giardina uses lunges to tone her hips and glutes.

Finish

Weighted Lunge

Weighted lunges bring your lower region more into play than the non-weighted or light weight lunge. The lunge is performed by standing straight up and then stepping far forward and down on one foot, leaving the other motionless in the initial spot. From this position you then push your body back up to the original standing spot. Performing this movement with weights (either a barbell across your back or with dumbells in your hands) will make the movement more difficult. And to overcome the difficulty the hips and buns will join in with more involvement, which in turn stimulates more muscle tone from both. As with the other weighted movements, gradually get used to the exercise and then slowly add

Your Fastest Way To A Sexy Butt

weight over the period of several weeks or months. Maintain good form by keeping your back straight throughout the movement.

Weighted Hip/Leg Raises

Hip/leg raises are done from a standing position. Slowly raise one of your legs out to the side of your body as high as possible. Hold this position for a second or so, then slowly lower it down back to the start. You can increase the efficacy of this exercise by using an ankle weight. An ankle weight makes it harder to complete the movement and you may not be able to hold your foot out to the side very long, but you will improve with time. Another version of this movement is performed with the ankle cable attachment, which works great as it keeps constant tension on the hip muscles. Repeat on both sides for several repetitions.

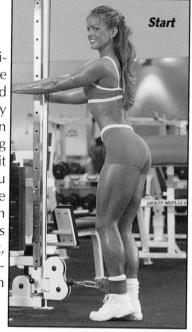

Start

Weighted Leg Raises to the Rear

This is a similar exercise to the previous one – use a low pulley cable with an ankle strap. Raise the leg (one at a time) to the rear, keeping the knee almost locked straight. Return until your foot is back alongside the non-exercising limb and repeat. Other than heavy squats this exercise works the upper glute muscle and helps to round out the buns better than any other exercise known. Repeat with the other leg.

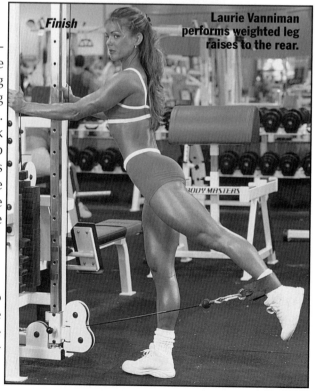

Finish

Laurie Vanniman performs weighted leg raises to the rear.

Repetition Range

The repetition range for bun/hip exercise directed at filling out the posterior can initially be lower since you will be using weights – heavier weights – more frequently. However,

Your Fastest Way To A Sexy Butt

try to get in at least eight repetitions per set. Use a similar set and repetition range, and workout frequency, as noted in the previous chapter.

Building up the Buns

You don't have to be stuck with flat buns or skinny hips if you use specific exercises to re-shape them. The exercises in this chapter will work very well toward adding some muscle tone and size and creating new contours to your posterior. The key to successfully building up some curves is to use weight in these various exercises. If you do so you can re-shape your posterior from flat and skinny into curvaceous and shapely.

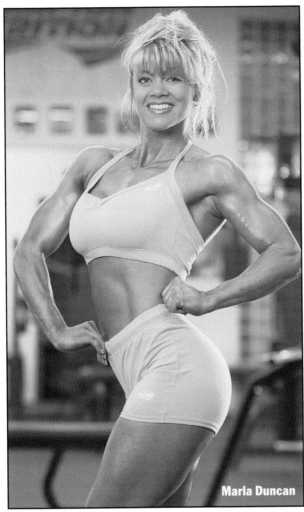

Marla Duncan

Summary

- Flat buns and skinny hips can be filled out through specific shaping exercises.
- The best exercise for filling out flat buns and skinny hips is the heavy squat.
- By using weights with a variety of the bun/hip exercises (squats, hyperextension, lunges, etc.) you can promote additional muscle size in the posterior region.

Chapter Three

TRIMMING FLABBY BUNS & HIPS

Trying to gain size in the backside is a problem that most women wish they had to deal with compared to the more frequent problem of flab. The most effective way to start trimming down is through specific shape exercise. Shape/strength exercise elevates the metabolism and this in turn burns bodyfat from all over the body, including the gluteal region. But shape/strength exercise is not the only tool that you have available for trimming down. There is another effective means for building lean and mean buns – aerobic exercise.

Specific Aerobic Exercise

Just as shape/strength exercise that is specific is far more effective, so too is aerobic exercise. All aerobic exercise will burn off bodyfat (provided you do it long enough) but not all aerobic exercise involves the same muscle groups. Some aerobic exercise such as rowing primarily involves the upper body. Other types of aerobic exercise such as running involve the legs more. By choosing specific types of aerobic exercise, you can double your gains when it comes to working on your glutes.

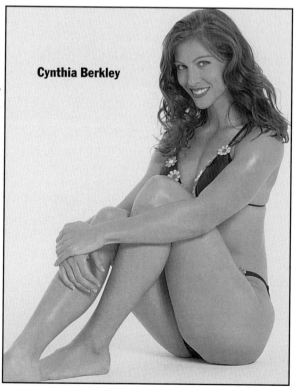

Cynthia Berkley

Your Fastest Way To A Sexy Butt

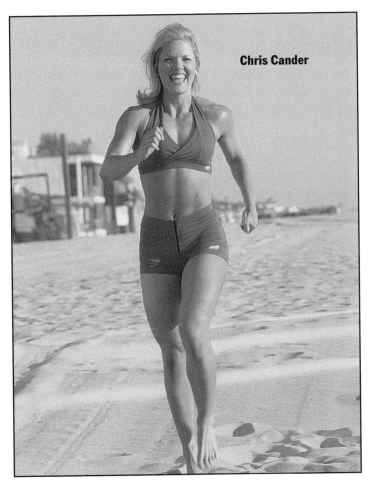

Chris Cander

Double Dipping

There are some aerobic exercises that utilize your gluteal muscles more in the action. By using these specific exercises you can get both the benefit of burning fat off as well as assisting in increasing the muscle tone of your hips and buns. This provides you with a "double-dip" from a single exercise.

What are the exercises that provide you with the dual benefits? These exercises include stair stepping, power walking, walking on the treadmill, motion aerobics (certain forms) and jogging. Each of these exercises gets the upper leg muscles more involved than other forms of aerobics. And if you have the chance to "double-dip" on your exercise benefits, it is always a good idea to take advantage of the situation. It will really help you shift your shape from flabby to firm much more quickly.

Your Fastest Way To A Sexy Butt

Combo Cardio/Aerobic Exercise

The exercises that provide the double benefits can be considered "combo" cardio/aerobic exercise. These exercises combine fat burning and cardio/respiratory benefits along with bun and hip shaping benefits. This combination greatly works to help you achieve your goals and emphasize use of the hips and buttocks. Stationary biking is an example of a lower body exercise that does not really have much direct involvement of your buns – because you are sitting on them, not using them! By avoiding the cardio/aerobic exercises that do not directly work your buttocks and hips and focusing instead on a specific type of exercise you can get the "combo" bene-fits for your buns and hips. By doing this you will get the standard benefit that all cardio/aerobic exercises provide – the overall loss of bodyfat (trimming down the hips and buns as part of the process). And you will also get some fantastic muscle toning benefits to boot – right in your buns!

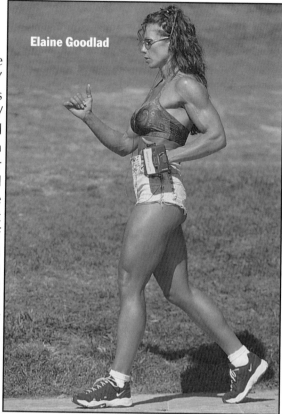

Elaine Goodlad

Power Walking

Power walking is a great exercise to burn off fat in general and it is a superb exercise for the buns and hips. The buns and hips move constantly in motoring your body around at a brisk clip. Power walking seems to use your bun and hip muscles even more than its cousin, jogging. Power walking, provided you do it at a brisk pace, is one of the very top bun/hip shaping exercises that you can use. The walking motion directly involves your buttocks and hips and you can make that involvement even more pronounced by contracting and relaxing your hips and buttocks repeatedly as you walk. Very few aerobic exercises allow you to directly contract the bun muscles in the midst of the workout like power walking does. Power walking is also ideal for burn-ing off bodyfat if you take longer walks (30+ minute range) on a consistent basis. Walking should be done at a fast clip (hence the name "power walking") to realize the full shaping potential of power walking.

Treadmill

If jogging is a close cousin to power walking, the treadmill is even closer. The treadmill is just about as good as power walking for bun and hip tightening. The treadmill has been touted as the "top gun" among indoor exercises as far as calorie burning is considered. And it is also tops for targeting the hip and bun muscles for some super shaping action. The treadmill keeps constantly coming at you as you exercise, forcing your fanny to get in a strong workout. You cannot "take it easy" on a treadmill – the track keeps coming at you continuously. And you can add emphasis to the treadmill session by contracting your buns tightly and then relaxing your contraction as you walk.

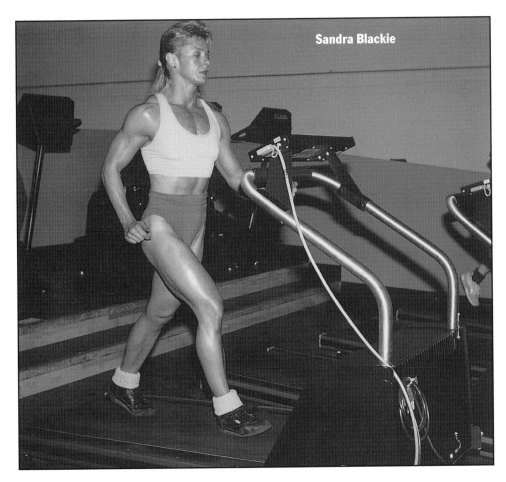

Sandra Blackie

Your Fastest Way To A Sexy Butt

Stair Stepping

Climbing stairs – any stairs, machine or on the real stairs – is a great "combo" exercise for forming firm buns and hips. The stepping action that you perform as you climb utilizes both the buns and hips on every step. Step after step you give your posterior a hard workout as you climb. The longer your climbing continues, the more bodyfat you burn off your physique. Climbing the stairs is a great choice for cardio/aerobic combo exercise. Vary the stair climbing stride that you use – generally the longer the stride, the more your tush is involved in the action.

You can add to the effect that stair climbing has on your buns by also climbing stairs at any and all opportunities besides the specific aerobic workout. Skip the elevator – take the stairs for better looking buns.

Step Aerobics

A close cousin of stair climbing is step aerobics. With step aerobics you also climb stairs except that it is singular, not plural – you step up and down on one platform instead of a machine or a staircase and you often do it to the beat of a jazzy tune. Since the same muscles (including the hips and buttocks) are used as for the stepping motion with step aerobics as with stair climbing, you also get the fat burning – muscle toning combo effect. And doing it to a musical beat can make your workout go quicker.

Motion Aerobics

Motion aerobic routines often incorporate stair climbing movements among the various motions as well. Sometimes a step is used in the session. And in addition to these climbing motions, motion aerobics also often utilizes exercises that involve specific "tightening" of the buns and hips such as mule kicks, etc.

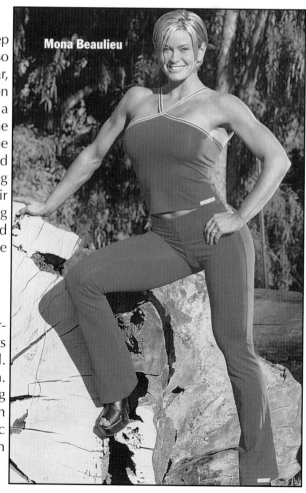

Mona Beaulieu

Your Fastest Way To A Sexy Butt

Jogging/Running

Jogging also gets your rear end heavily involved in propelling your body along and therefore is also a good combo cardio/aerobic exercise. If you use this exercise, make certain to jog or run on surfaces that have some "give" as hard surfaces such as concrete can cause injuries to your legs and joints.

Combo Cardio/aerobic Exercises

Choose one of these "combo" cardio/aerobic exercises and use it consistently to get the dual benefits of burning fat off your body and shaping up your physique. There are a variety of good cardio/ aerobic exercises but these that have been featured in this chapter are the best if you are aiming at changing the shape of your posterior.

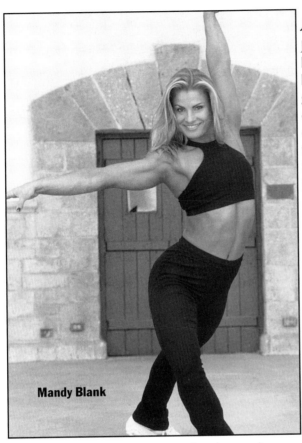

Mandy Blank

Perform your "combo" cardio/aerobic workout two to five times a week (depending upon what your weekly schedule allows) for 20 minutes or more of non-stop action. If possible, go for longer cardio/aerobic sessions (30-45 minutes) for quicker and more significant results.

You are not stuck with performing the same "combo" cardio/aerobic exercise all of the time. Don't get caught in a routine rut as one of the main enemies of training consistency can rear its head – boredom. Beat the boredom problem by alternating the various combo cardio/aerobic exercises instead of using the same old routine again and again. Use power walking on one day, jogging on another, and stair stepping on yet another day. Or use several sessions of the same exercise and then switch to a different "combo" cardio/aerobic exercise for the next few workouts. But always include one of these hot combo exercises if you want the multiple benefits they provide.

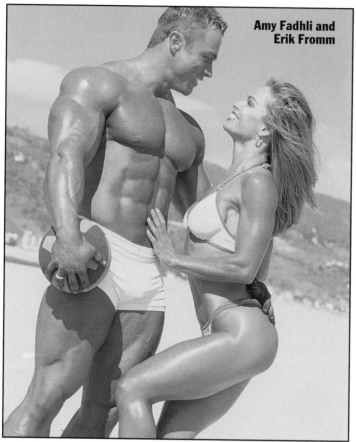

Amy Fadhli and
Erik Fromm

Fighting Bun Flab

One dictionary definition of flab is "loose, unwanted fatty tissue on the body". As unwanted as fat is, it is even more undesirable in your hips and buttocks. Flab in this area can cause havoc with the overall appearance of the physique, expanding the appearance of your posterior.

One of the best tools for fighting flab and burning it off the body is cardio/aerobic exercise because cardio/aerobic exercise uses fat as the primary fuel source for the workout. And the longer the workout lasts (beyond the 20 minute mark), the more flab is burned off the body. When done consistently, cardio/aerobic exercise will carve the unwanted flab off and to reveal the nice contours underneath. If you use the specific cardio/aerobic exercises that readily utilize the gluteal muscles during the action, these "combo" exercises will hasten the process of shaping those contours. So get into the "combo" cardio/aerobic exercises for the shape you want and deserve.

Summary

- Cardio/aerobic exercise uses bodyfat for the primary fuel source as the workout progresses beyond 20 minutes of non-stop action.
- Certain cardio/aerobic exercises such as power walking, jogging, the treadmill, stair climbing and motion aerobics provide a combination effect of burning off fat and shaping the muscle tone of the buttocks.
- The more frequently you perform these combo cardio/aerobic exercises the quicker you will win the war against flab.

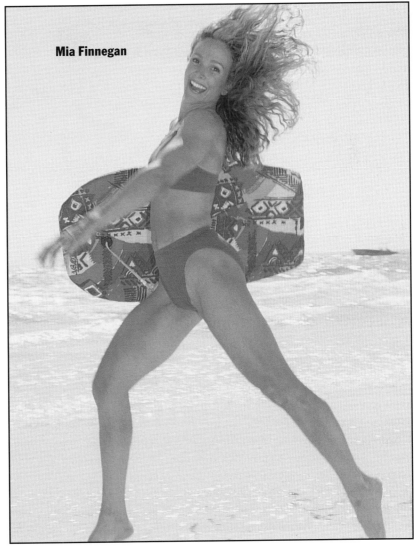

Mia Finnegan

Your Fastest Way To A Sexy Butt

Chapter Four

EXTRA CREDIT

Most people are familiar with the concept of extra credit in school terminology. Often a teacher or instructor will allow the students to do some extra work for extra points that count toward the final grade. Extra credit is a handy way to improve your position. The same is true for building your physique. You can supplement your training with a few "extra credit" techniques that will help hasten the bun and hip shaping process. These extra credit items will help you get the inside track in taking control of the condition of your posterior. By mixing them with the other elements of specific shape training and "combo" cardio/aerobic exercise, you will get to where you want to go with your rear shape quicker.

Pro-Active Attack

A major problem that many people face in trimming and tightening the bun/hip area is the sedentary lifestyle that most people live. Not only does this lifestyle that most of the population (close to 70 percent of the US, according to some physicians) engage in contribute to poor health – it is also the major factor for the poor shape of the average person's physique. Your hips and buttocks are not exempt from this problem – if anything, they are more at risk since they tend to accumulate fat more quickly. Sedentary living can be devastating to your health. Aerobic trainer and television fitness star Denise Austin noted this problem in stating that "sitting is the worst thing for your buns". Unfortunately, that is exactly what most people do – sit. If you think about it most people sit a lot. They sit at work, sit on the drive home, sit to eat and then come home and sit in front of the television. Surveys of viewing habits indicate that most people spend several hours in front of the television every day – sitting or reclining. This spreading out in front of the television leads to calling out the fat brigade as the body's metabolism slows way down. To make matters worse, food is often one of the main staples while the television is viewed. The amount of snack food sold increased by 1.4 billion pounds between 1987 and 1996. These extra calories are going somewhere – on your physique. As people "super-size it" on their menu, they in turn are unwittingly "supersizing" their hips and buns. Slowly but steadily extra weight is added to the body, and more than a fair share ends up on your rear end.

Kim Hartt

What is the best way to address this problem of the sedentary lifestyle and the weight problem generated by the increased intake of large amounts of food? The best way is to become pro-active and attack back. People who are reactive tend to use danger-ous tools such as dietary drugs (remember Phen-fen and Redux?) to respond to the problem. But the best approach is not to react but to be proactive. Don't just sit there on your buns and let them get bigger! Aerobic trainer Denise Austin provides a fabulous example of how to fight back. She is very active almost all of the time, not sitting down but standing, walking, and moving. In an article in *Self Employed*, she points out that one of her tips for staying in shape is to move around, even when she is on phone calls. Denise models the premier manner in which to meet the encroachment of sedentary size gains – become more pro-active by physical activity. Instead of letting fat subtly accumulate around your buns and hips uncontended, fight back by becoming more active in your daily lifestyle.

Your Fastest Way To A Sexy Butt

Becoming more active during the day (particularly on a consistent basis) assists your body in shaping a tighter and trimmer hip/buttock area in two ways. Your "active" movement will utilize your hip and buttock muscles and help tone them (the more you walk, the more they work), and your more active lifestyle will increase your metabolic rate, moving it to a higher level. This increase in the metabolic rate (from the more active lifestyle you are now living) in turn burns off fat.

Use it or lose it

Muscles that are not used consistently shrink and become weaker (atrophy). If you are in the habit of sitting around all of the time with your primary activity a trip to the refrigerator for some more goodies, you will not utilize the full potential of the muscles of your hips and buttocks. Walking is one of the very best ways to work these muscles, and the more of it you do, the better your butt will appear. People with a more active lifestyle tend to have tighter and trimmer hips and buttocks than those who are more sedentary. And it does not take that much effort to increase your daily activity level. Start walking more. Take the stairs. Stand instead of sit. You get the idea – move around!

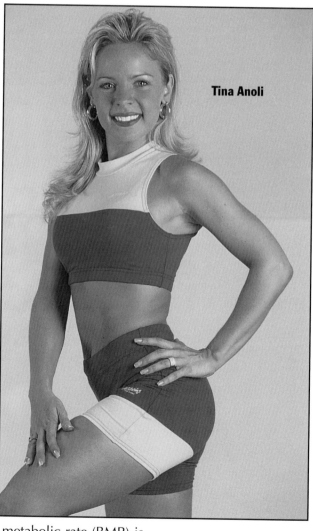

Tina Anoli

Metabolic Burn

As you move around more frequently you not only get exercise but you also increase your body's overall metabolic rate. Your basal metabolic rate (BMR) is one vital area when it comes to winning the war with fat. The control of your physique's metabolic rate is one of the premier factors in trimming fat off your physique. Dr. Dennis Sparkman, has pointed out (August 1997 issue of

Your Fastest Way To A Sexy Butt

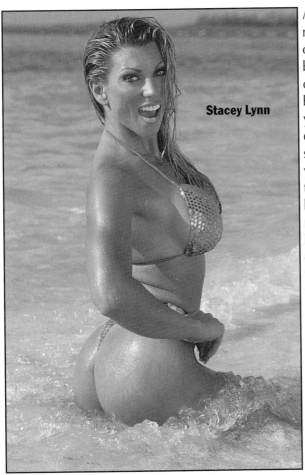

Stacey Lynn

Men's Workout) that "one of our main reasons for wanting to increase our BMR is that it is responsible for burning 60 to 75 percent of all the calories used by the body on a daily basis". Nothing affects the fat level of your physique like your metabolism does – particularly when it is responsible for most of the calories that your body burns. If you want to take total control when it comes to your bodyfat level, then aim at using your metabolism. And this control of your bodyfat level via your metabolism is especially important in relation to your bun/hip region. Since much of the fatty weight that most women gain goes on to the hip/buttock area, when fat is burned it will tend to come off these same areas. Your metabolic rate is a key factor for fat loss all over your body, and it is a key element for fat loss in the posterior section of your physique. In fact, it is the most important element. As pointed out previously, your metabolism makes up the major portion, 60 to 75 percent, of your body's caloric burning activity. The higher your metabolism, the more calories you burn each day. It is basically that simple. And many of the calories that get burned off are from your bodyfat stores. Your basal metabolic rate plays a major role in how many calories per hour you burn, so use it to your advantage by "hyping" it with more activity.

How does this work? A portion of your metabolic rate is hereditary, and a portion of it is influenced by your daily personal choices. Someone who comes home and watches the TV for hours a night while snacking on junk food consistently will be lowering their base metabolic rate while someone who comes home and works around the house for a few hours in the evening habitually will be raising their basal metabolic rate. Activity is a fantastic tool to use to burn off unwanted body fat. This is true in nature – the cheetah is much trimmer than the sloth; the shark is

Your Fastest Way To A Sexy Butt

trimmer than the seal – and it works in human action also. Activity requires fuel, and some of the fuel is bodyfat. As your base metabolic rate climbs higher it will burn off more fat throughout the day. The fat that the body burns off comes from all over the body, but for women most it will come from where the most is stored – around the hip and buttock regions. This in turn plays a tremendously large role in whether or not you have flabby rolls around your hips and buttocks. The more active you are on a consistent basis, the higher your metabolic rate and the more fat you burn off your buns and hips.

Genetics and Choice

Some people are blessed with a more active metabolism and have a higher basal

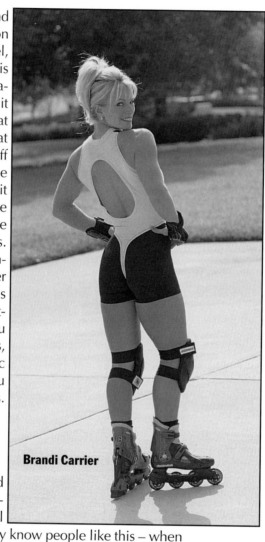

Brandi Carrier

metabolic rate. You probably know people like this – when they are younger this allows them to eat a lot of food without gaining and ounce of fat. It is simply a matter of being born with a higher metabolic rate. Is it equitable that some people are born with such a super physical advantage? No, but who said life was fair? If you have a higher metabolism you will have an easier time keeping fat off of your physique. If not, you will need to take a different path to slimming your body.

Those who are fortunate to be born with a higher metabolic rate often find that their metabolism starts to slow down as they start to get older, making it harder to stay trim – even for them. That's the bad news. But there is good news. The good news is that you are not stuck at the

Your Fastest Way To A Sexy Butt

same metabolic rate forever. Your genetics are not the only factor in the game. You can choose to do some things that will increase your metabolic rate. And when you do these things on a habitual basis, you will be able to unconsciously burn off bodyfat.

You can start to influence your metabolic rate (hype it) by moving away from sedentary living to a more active lifestyle. This does not mean that you have to literally run everywhere, but you can walk a lot more frequently than what you are currently doing. Take the stairs instead of always using the elevator. Aim at keeping your body moving more frequently and for longer time periods. When you start to become aware of your daily activity habits you will find many ways that you can move about more often and more vigorously. Anyone can benefit from the accumulation of moderate physical activity, even if it occurs in short, scattered periods outside of formal exercise programs. These "scattered periods" of physical activity effectively elevate your metabolism. The majority of people are sedentary and by switching to an active lifestyle they can make some significant changes in the shape of their physique (as well as in the area of health). By moving about more actively and frequently you can boost your metabolism and cause more calories to be burned off. It is very simple to do – just sit and lay down less, and "move your buns" more often. The more frequently you "move your buns", the more fat you will lose – fat that comes off from all over and particularly from around your buns and hips.

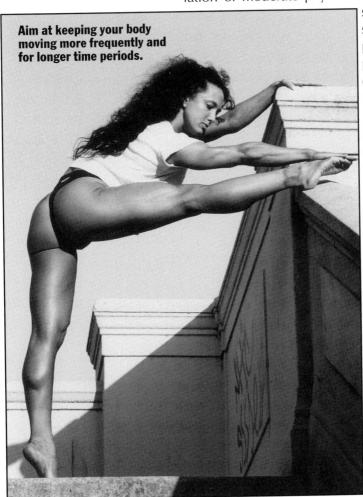

Aim at keeping your body moving more frequently and for longer time periods.

Your Fastest Way To A Sexy Butt

The Food Factor

There is one other major factor when it comes to shaping your glutes – the food factor. Your diet directly contributes to the condition of your buns and hips.

The first step in handling your diet is to prevent it from putting on any more unwanted flab. Many people find it a tough go to get the body to give up fat once it is stored in the buns and hips. So prevention of any further accumulation is the first step forward.

The best thing that you can do is to reduce the number of calories that you are eating each day. This sounds simple, but many people ignore this area. You cannot afford to overlook your caloric intake if you want hot hips and buns. Any excess, whether excess fat, carbohydrates, or even protein, is stored by the body as fat. You have to be especially careful with fat intake since it has more than twice the calories per gram that protein and carbohydrates do. Fat is not the only culprit when it comes to gaining unwanted weight. If you eat more protein or carbohydrates than your body needs, they will be stored as fat. You have to be careful with carbohydrates because even though they do not have as many calories per gram as fat, they add up quickly. This is particularly true of food items that contain sugar. It does not take a lot of sugar to add up to a lot of calories.

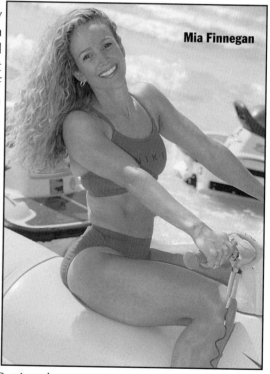

Mia Finnegan

Cutting back on caloric intake should be done gradually. If you suddenly stop eating, your metabolism will slow down drastically. And that is exactly what you do not want to happen. In addition to not cutting out your calories too fast, don't cut back on your calories too far – your body needs some calories for the energy necessary to get through the day and for adequate nutrition. Cutting down on calories too soon and too much will actually work against your desire to lose fat. When you drop your caloric intake to virtually nothing your metabolism also drops down rapidly – short-circuiting what you are trying to do. And you don't want your metabolism to slow down because that is the most powerful fat-fighting tool that you

Your Fastest Way To A Sexy Butt

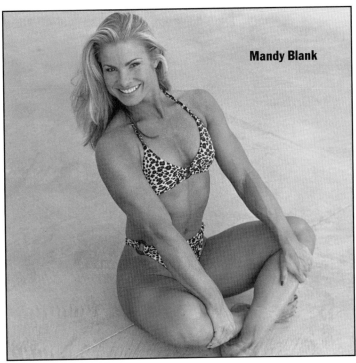

Mandy Blank

have. So cut back on calorie levels at a gradual pace. Make it your aim to slowly "curb" rather than drastically cut your calories.

Week 1
Cut out 50 calories per day (total weekly reduction of 350 calories).

Week 2
Cut out 75 calories per day (total weekly reduction of 525 calories)

Week 3
Cut out 100 calories per day (total weekly reduction of 700 calories).

Week 4
Cut out 125 calories per day (total weekly reduction of 875 calories).

At this point (having cut back on your normal caloric intake by 125 calories per day) assess where you are at. Are you getting enough calories for daily energy needs? Considering that you are expending more calories with the shape/strength exercise and the aerobic exercise, are you at the right calories level? A good caloric level to be at is one where you are losing fat but still have a lot of energy for activities. You do not need to make huge changes in your caloric level if you are exercising with both shape/strength workouts and aerobic workouts, as well as increasing your daily activity levels. Each of these will act to assist your body in trimming down and makes extreme dietary changes unnecessary.

If you do find that you need to lose more fat, continue to gradually cut back on your calories. Pay close attention to what you eat and slowly taper it off.

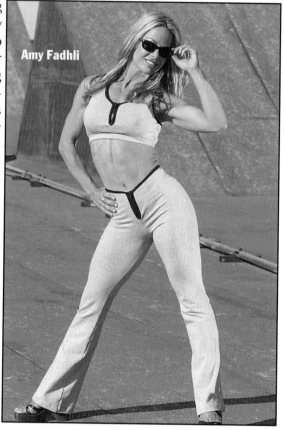

Amy Fadhli

Week 5
Cut out 150 calories per day (total weekly reduction of 1,050 calories).

Week 6
Cut out 175 calories per day (total weekly reduction of 1,225 calories).

Week 7
Cut out 200 calories per day (total weekly reduction of 1,400 calories).

Week 8
Cut out 225 calories per day (total weekly reduction of 1,575 calories).

Again assess your progress. You may be moving into a caloric plateau – a place where you can allow your eating to level off. The best way to check your fat loss progress is with a combination of a tape measure, fat caliper, weight scale, and the mirror. None of these alone is enough to make a good judgement, but together they team up to give you a good idea of your progress. The tape measure is not a total answer because you may lose an inch of fat while gaining an inch of muscle – giving you

Your Fastest Way To A Sexy Butt

good progress even though the tape measure remains the same. Or you may think you have only lost three pounds in two months of exercise when you actually have lost nine pounds of fat and gained six pounds of lean, toned muscle. So use each of the checking elements together to find out how you are doing. And also consider your energy level. Leave enough calories in your diet to give you the daily energy to continue functioning at peak levels.

Some people may find that they still need to cut out more calories. Although many people can cut down on only a small amount of calories and see results (when combined with exercise), the fat may fight to stay on for others. In this case continue to slowly reduce the calorie intake level.

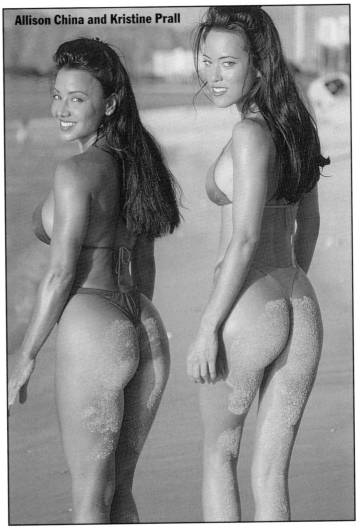

Allison China and Kristine Prall

Your Fastest Way To A Sexy Butt

Week 9

Cut out 250 calories per day (total weekly reduction of 1,750).

Week 10

Cut out 275 calories per day (total weekly reduction of 1,925 calories).

Week 11

Cut out 300 calories per day (total weekly reduction of 2,100 calories).

Week 12

Cut out 325 calories per day (total weekly reduction of 2,275 calories).

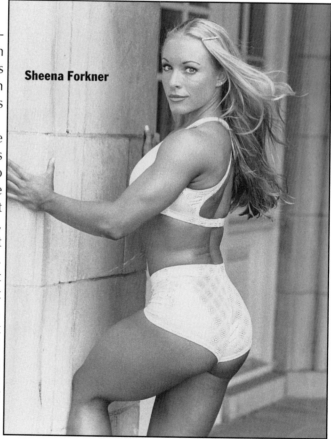

Sheena Forkner

Slowly reduce the calories until you get those trim contours in the hips and buns that you want. Mix exercise with caloric reduction to make things happen.

The sources that you use for obtaining your calories is important. It is not a good idea to eat a lot of sugar and fat (the typical person's diet). Instead, eat more fresh fruits, vegetables, quality low-fat protein, low-fat milk products, and lots of fiber. Eat more grains – whole wheat instead of refined flour. Eat oatmeal instead of sugary cereal. Eat nuts and seeds for your fat instead of pastries. Use olive oil or canola for cooking. By making a few changes you can greatly upgrade the nutrition level of your diet and enhance the appearance of your physique.

Eating right not only helps you keep the unwanted fat off your body, it also gives you the right nutrients that you need to sustain your body in daily living. Your body needs certain "essential elements" and it is crucial that you

Your Fastest Way To A Sexy Butt

get them to avoid any of a variety of illnesses and diseases. When you reduce your caloric intake it is more important than ever that the food that you do eat is very nutritious and provides your body with a variety of the essential elements. So skip the junk food and eat nutritiously – for both your appearance and your health. And by doing this habitually you will also assist your progress in shaping your buns and hips.

You can give your glute shaping program a strong boost by becoming more active during the day and by controlling your diet. Each of these important areas can strongly contribute to your goal of building a great derriere in a positive way so don't neglect them. Move more, eat less.

Summary

- Move around more frequently. One of the main contributing factors to a fat and unhealthy physique is a sedentary lifestyle.
- Your metabolism is the main element in burning off body fat. Increase your metabolism by becoming more active every day.
- Assist your bun/hip shaping effort by cutting back on your caloric intake.
- Gradually cut your caloric intake. Curb your calorie intake rather than drastically cutting it.
- Sitting is not good for your glute shape. Stand and move more often.

Shape Your Buns and Hips

Give yourself some time as you use these bun/hip shaping elements. Don't expect to radically re-shape your posterior in ten days. Aim at a few months instead of a few days, and you will take the pressure off of yourself and your workout program. The best change is that which remains for the long term, and by approaching your training in a gradual manner you give yourself the inside track to shaping success. Whether your buns and hips are too flabby or too flat, you can change the way they look. Use the direction in this book to guide you down the path to a slim and shapely posterior.

Your Fastest Way To A Sexy Butt

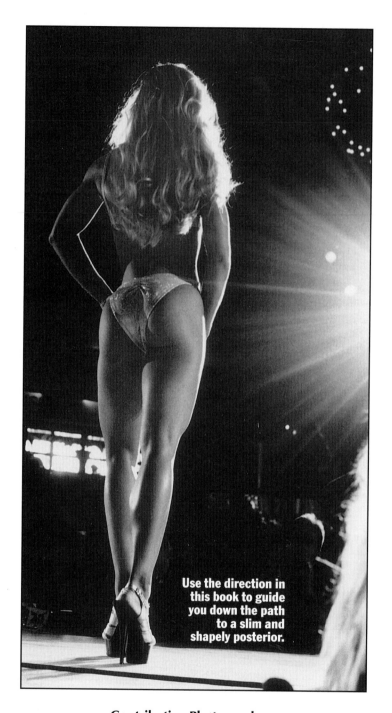

Use the direction in this book to guide you down the path to a slim and shapely posterior.

Contributing Photographers

Jim Amentler, Alex Ardenti, Reg Bradford, Ralph DeHaan,
Skip Faulkner, Irvin Gelb, Robert Kennedy, Jason Mathas,
Rob Sims, Art Zeller